# YOUR KNOWLEDGE HAS VALUE

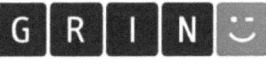

# Exploring the Role of Positive Psychology in Burnout among Nursing Professionals

Akinmayowa Adedoyin Shobo

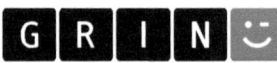

**Bibliographic information published by the German National Library:**

The German National Library lists this publication in the National Bibliography; detailed bibliographic data are available on the Internet at http://dnb.dnb.de.

ISBN: 9783346573810
This book is also available as an ebook.

© GRIN Publishing GmbH
Nymphenburger Straße 86
80636 München

Print and binding: Books on Demand GmbH, Norderstedt, Germany
Printed on acid-free paper from responsible sources.

The present work has been carefully prepared. Nevertheless, authors and publishers do not incur liability for the correctness of information, notes, links and advice as well as any printing errors.

GRIN web shop: https://www.grin.com/document/1165281

# Exploring the Role of Positive Psychology in Burnout among Nursing Professionals

**2021**

# Table of Content

## Abstract

Stress appears to be a normal response to certain agency that requires the application of our capabilities to adapt to changing environmental conditions. In the care of patients, the working environment typically encompass well-defined structures such as healthcare institutions (regardless of their levels of expertise) or informal settings commonly found in many resource-limited settings where access to formal institutions may be temporarily or permanently unavailable.

The present work focuses on the subject of burn-out among nursing professionals owing to a myriad of factors. It highlights the phenomena of stress in the workplace and individual's lives of nurses; existing assumptions on burnout as an indicator of stress and its mechanistic pathways within a health organization. This is followed by literature analysis of research works on the impact of burnout, in particular, as barrier to achieving the ultimate goal of quality and safe patient care and the role of positive psychology.

In sum, it is imperative that the promotion of health and the prevention of health problems (particularly among nurses) should majorly be focused on creating a work environment that does not induce an unnecessary amount of stress and that can compensate for unavoidable stress in the form of increased control and rewards for workers among other incentives.

## Introduction: The Concept of Stress

The term 'stress' hardly has a general consensus in its meaning among various researchers. Several arguments have been put forward as described below. McGrath (1976) (cited in Moustaka & Constantinidis, 2010) argued that stress ensues when a person perceives a high demand on their personal capabilities from the environment. Such high expectation and demand may elicit fear reactions and stress. Williams and Huber (1986) theory in a way supports this argument viewing the persistent high demand of one's capabilities as akin to the perception of threat from internal or external sources in a particular circumstance. Arnold and Feldman (1986) posits that such 'stressful' response is individual-dependent. French *et al.* (1985) postulates on the indiscriminate nature of stress – the phenomenon of stimulating a response (either burn-out or rust-out) "...when we surpass our limitations or we are below them" as we exhibit our capabilities in the presence of a 'threat' or challenging situation.

In short, the sources of the 'threat' will be addressed subsequently as it concerns the workplace (in this case, the healthcare institutions).

## Concept of Stress and Burn-out

There is a widely accepted assumption that individuals at some point (either in their personal or professional lives) would have to face conditions that are geared to enhance their performance, capabilities and general quality of life (Tehrani & Ayling, 2009). On the other hand, there are also awareness on setbacks to personal and professional life brought by inability to manage the stress levels within the environment, often manifesting as "...loss of productivity and working hours, development of diseases, workplace accidents among others" (Lazarus and Folkman, 1984 cited in Moustaka & Constantinidis, 2010). Researchers have exposed some of the negative responses to stress to include gastric ulcer, hypertension, asthma, heart attack, anxiety, burnout, amnesia and fussiness to mention a few (Tehrani et al., 2012).

As indicated earlier, as individual enter various transition in their personal and professional lives; they encounter threats, unfamiliar events or challenges that Matteson and Ivancevich (1987) (in Kumari and Mishra, 2009) identified as stressors or stress-causing agents. Their response to these stressors therefore is what is perceived as stress. It has also been described as a reaction to "...

6

change in the environment which is often associated with danger, challenge or threat to an individual's stable condition" (Smeltzer *et al.*, 2008; Gorgich *et al.*, 2017).

Although this discourse is focused on the nurse as a professional; various studies have demonstrated how an individual's personal life is inextricably linked to their capabilities to manage stress at the workplace. Conceptually, there is a relationship between "health, relationship and financial challenges on the home front, and being able to cope with the demands of patient care, and other external forces in their work environment" (Bromberger & Matthews, 1996; Rothmann, Van Der Colff, & Rothmann, 2006). Understanding this relationship is pivotal to addressing the consequent outcomes of poor stress management decisions perceived as "… burnout, job satisfaction and health outcomes through a pattern of physiological, emotional, behavioural and cognitive processes" (Young, Schieman & Milkie, 2013).

The next section is focused on stress in the working environment of nurses.

## Stress and Nursing Professionals

Having a robust health workforce is a significant indication of a strong health system, and to a large extent, the performance of a health organization is predicated on collective state of the capacities of individuals that make up the health workforce (Kumari & Mishra, 2009). There are therefore, increasing calls for policies that ensure that health administrators and managers provide optimum working conditions for employees as a way of bolstering their productivity.

Kumari and Mishra (2009) worked on "...identifying stress-related factors that positively and negatively affect performance of medical professionals." Their report indicated some of the common stressors that affect many individuals particularly in clinical or non-clinical environments such as "... overload, role conflict, and general lack of clarity in job specifications." Meanwhile, contrarily to overwhelming assumptions, stressors may either present as opportunities or barriers to the growth of individuals. In other words, positive stress present individuals with opportunities for having or doing what they desire. Negative stress on the other hand, is characterized by overwhelming and undesirable barriers or demands on the individual. This is otherwise known as *distress* in certain literature (Ravalier *et al.*, 2020).

Most workplace stress have been profiled in scholarly works such that undesirable work-related conditions are found to be unintentionally or innately created leading to transformation in the health status of individuals, "...reinforcing deviation from normal functioning" (Beehr & Newman, 1978).

Distress in the workplace as defined by the United Kingdom Health and Safety Executive (HSE) is "the adverse reaction individuals have to excessive pressures or other demands placed on them" (Ravalier *et al.*, 2020).

There are many sources of stress for healthcare providers including stress associated with providing care to patients (Kabirzadeh *et al.*, 2008); when stress become persistent, it could lead to the phenomenon known as "physical and mental burnout (Gorgich *et al.*, 2017). This is in agreement with Beddoe and Murphy (2004) that found the work-related stress can increasingly affect worker's mental and physical health. It is also consistent with studies by Piko (2006) and Khamisa *et al.* (2016) that correlated poor physical and psychological health outcomes with work-related stress and burnout.

Ravalier, McVicar and Boichat (2020) study characterised workplace stress among employees of the National Health Service (NHS) based on the background of "higher-than-average level of stress-related sickness absence of all jobs sectors in the country." From the study, it was reported that the health and social care occupational sectors had the highest levels of stress-related sickness absence in the country, estimated to be 46% higher than the United Kingdom (UK) average (Rimmers, 2018). Of this statistics, job-related stress leading to poor health outcomes accounted for approximately 40% of absenteeism (Rimmer, 2018); consequently, leading to financial losses of "…up to £400 million" annually (NHS, 2020).

In the discourse on distress ensuing from fulfilling the overwhelming physical and mental demands of the workplace, it is important to acknowledge why the subject is important for the healthcare professional (notably, the nurse) who is typically confronted by a myriad of hazards that threaten their health, as defined by the World Health Organisation (WHO). The WHO definition typically expands the health of individuals in multidimensional fashion including physical, mental and social (Behrouzian *et al.*, 2009; Samiee *et al.*, 2011).

In recent times, many public debates have been centred on allocation of financial resources to create the ideal work environment for health workers and the expected dividends (Lu, Chang & Lu, 2007). The health statistics on budgetary allocation for such purposes that reflects the conditions of the working environment is often reported to be worse in resource-limited countries such as in sub-Saharan Africa.

As noted by Gorgich and other researchers, nurses due to their role in the health system are highly impacted by the stressful work environment compared to other professionals" (Gorgich *et al.*, 2017). In fact, they are estimated to constitute a high demand of approximately 80% of the healthcare providers (Ghasemi & Attar, 2008).

Meanwhile, the WHO in one of its reports ranked nursing professionals high in terms of health problems (risks to occupational hazards) - "...27 out of 130 stressful jobs" (Sepehrmanesh *et al.*, 2003).

Further, based on the extensive empirical studies of the effect of burn-out and other distress signs on nurses; a number of contributory elements to raise the potential for burnout among nurses have been identified including "...working environment, interpersonal relationship, role characteristics among others" (Moustaka and Constantinidis, 2010; Gorgich *et al.*, 2017; Khamisa *et al.*, 2017). This is as depicted in table 1 below.

# Table 1: Sources of Burn-out among nurses

| Research subject (sources of burn-out) | Research findings | References |
|---|---|---|
| **Working environment** | Difficulties in coping with stress combined with psychological or emotional instability; risk of physical violence, particularly in the emergency rooms constitute source of stress | Gray-Toft and Adderson (1981); Cooper (1978) |
| **Interpersonal Relationship** | Conflicts with co-workers, negative effect of lack of understanding and support from their managers are termed stress sources | Sveinsdottir *et al.* (2006); Health and Safety Executive (2020) |
| **Nature of nursing** | Unrealistic career expectations; strenuous work demands due to shortage of employees; being in a constantly emotional charged atmosphere such as the death of patients; occupational accident such as needle prick and contact with infectious agents | Hudgins, 2008; Cooper (1998); Bouvet (2007) |
| **Organizational factors** | Organizational and management framework; increased job demands, Inappropriate communications, introduction of new technologies, lack of task autonomy and feedback, career advancement, rising workload; budget cuts; transition in health care from hospital-based services to primary and community based services, having to deal with larger population. | Santos *et al.* (2003); Jennings, 2007; Koen *et al.*, (2011) |
| **Role characteristics** | Ambiguity or lack of clarity in job specification leading to low job satisfaction; lack of job opportunities for nurse (professionalism); lack of positive feedback from patients; feelings of inadequacy; redundancy | Sveinsdottir *et al.*, 2006; Aiken *et al.*, 2001; Moustaka *et al.*, 2009; Williams & Smith, 2013; Graham *et al.*, 2011; Moustaka & Constantinidis, 2010 |
| **Individual characteristics** | Lack of preparedness leading anxiety; lack of professional experience and education; A review by Khamisa *et al.* (2017) highlighted the interconnectedness between personal and work stress among nurses revealed that poor management of work-life balance often lead to mental health disorders such as depression. | Sveinsdottir *et al.*, 2006; Lee and Wang, 2002; Killien, 2004 |

It is important to note that addressing these above enlisted conditions that elicit negative stress response could help prevent adverse outcomes of burnout on the well-being of nurses (Gorgich et al., 2017; Shakerinia & Mohammadpour, 2010). This has been revealed based on the rate of "... sickness, high turnover, medical errors, presenteeism, absenteeism, intentions to leave the profession... among others" (Moustaka & Constantinidis, 2010; Houdmont, 2016; Ravalier et al., 2020).

Khamisa and co-researchers (2017) aptly delineated the typical pathway that leads to burnout using the Maslach's Burnout Model. The model has been used to explain the relationship between personal, job-related stress, burnout, job satisfaction and general health of nurses. I represented the interactions between these variables in figure 1 below. In similar manner, another approach to understanding how burn-out among nurses ensues is depicted in the job demands–resources (JDR) model (Bakker et al., 2013). The model postulates that "... resources act as buffer against job demands. However, if a condition is created where job demands outweigh the resources available, the outcome is burnout and distress" (Schaufeli et al., 2004; 2009, in Khamisa et al., 2017).

In a study by Khamisa *et al.* (2017) aimed at investigating whether personal stress is a more significant predictor of burnout, job satisfaction and general health than work-related stress. Findings revealed that "… personal stress is a better predictor of burnout and general health than job satisfaction which is better predicted by work stress." This, in a way, alludes to the contributory role of the personal lives of nursing professionals in their performance as nurses.

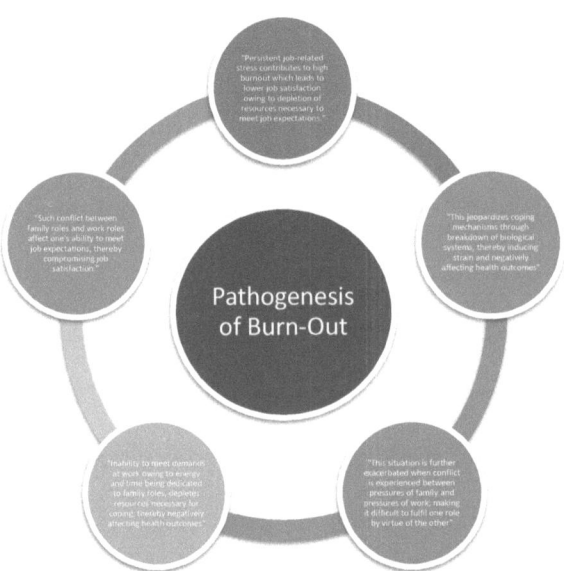

**Figure 1: Pathogenesis of Burn-out** (Source: Khamisa *et al.*, 2017, remodified by the author of this work)

As such, it is highly imperative to conduct research and develop policies that can help mitigate the costs of burn-out among nurses, which can cause distress on quality of health service delivery. Several studies have highlighted how such stress (irrespective of the source) perpetuate poor clinical services (Samadi *et al.*, 2013). Therefore, some of the approaches that have been suggested include "... reducing responsibilities, time flexibility, coordinating the job and individual's ability and programs for better quality of life would lead to stress reduction and enhance job satisfaction (Sepehrmanesh *et al.*, 2013).

Additionally, other solutions to mitigating cases of burn-out have also been proffered. For instance; "...where the level of job ambiguity is significant, there has been suggestions to re-present the vision and mission to employees" (Flaherty *et al.*, 1999, in Gorgich *et al.*, 2017). It may also be helpful to integrate staff trainings (nurses particularly) on organizational mission and objectives in a bid to optimize performance while resolving the lack of clarity in job description (Gorgich *et al.*, 2017).

This next section is aimed at evaluating the effectiveness of positive psychology, as a stress management instrument at the workplace.

**Perspectives on Stress Management Interventions (SMI)**

In various studies; workplace stress has been linked to a whole range of harmful physiological, psychological and behavioral reactions to situations (Mohammad, 2014; Katic *et al.*, 2019). Certain researchers have argued that an individual with a lower stress level tend to exhibit higher job satisfaction and are generally more inclined to be more productive in organisations (Siegrist, 2008; Fried, 2013).

There has been various works on workplace stress, notably those based on the transactional model of stress (Lazarus and Launier, 1978; Escartín *et al.*, 2009; Popov and Popov, 2011) which takes into account the well-being of an individual and an organization, particularly its financial goals and social responsibility.

Katic *et al.* (2019) postulated that sources of work stress (stressors) may be *individual* - arising from the work role; *group* - caused by the group's dynamics and managers' behavior; or *organizational* - arising from the organization's characteristics. Another model held that the tasks an employee has to perform (job demands) and the perceived degree of control he holds over the job demands (job control) may account for a certain degree of stress at work. For instance; there are studies that suggest that the highest amount of stress at work is expected in situations with high demands and low control (Karasek, 1979).

Today, there are increasing evidence that shows that stress at work, especially when chronic, constitute a risk to psychological and physical health of individuals and their organisations as reported in Ivancevich *et al.* (1990) and Berber and Lekovic (2018). As such, it is imperative that the promotion of health and the prevention of health problems should majorly be focused on creating a work environment that does not induce an unnecessary amount of stress and that can compensate for unavoidable stress in the form of increased control and rewards for workers (Bickford, 2005; Melchior *et al.*, 2008; Nelson & Simmons, 2011).

In a bid to mitigate the challenges of workplace stress, experts have been able to distinguish the roles diverse forms of stress perception (that is, *distress* and *eustress*) can play in the organization. Accordiingly, researchers have highlighted the importance of reducing distress at the workplace while promoting eustress; often referred to a positive form of stress that nurtures a more productive and conducive working environment (Nelson and Cooper, 2007; Nelson and Simmons, 2011; Kurpiyanov and Zhdanov, 2014).

Stress as widely accepted is a normal occurrence in life. To this end, individuals (and organisations) may not be able completely eliminate stress. Perhaps this is the reason why today, there's growing attention for adopting stress management programs to reduce the distress levels of their workforce. Some of the currently employed intervention are designed for instance; to change the organization of work in terms of *task characteristics, work conditions*, and *social aspects* (Semmer, 2006)

In another way, interventions at workplace have been suggested for appropriation at primary, secondary, or tertiary levels. Briefly, the *primary interventions* attempt to alter the sources of stress at work - for example; redesigning jobs to modify workplace stressors, increasing workers' decision-making authority; or providing co-worker support groups (Bond and Bunce, 2000; Murphy and Sauter, 2004). In contrast, *secondary interventions* are targeted at reducing the severity of stress symptoms before they lead to serious health problems (Murphy and Sauter, 2004). Meanwhile, the *tertiary interventions* such as employee assistance programs are designed to treat the employee's health condition via free and confidential access to qualified mental health professionals (Arthur, 2000).

Accordingly, the most common interventions are the ones particularly target the individual which involves instructions in managing and coping with stress (Giga *et al.*, 2003). These include cognitive–behavioral skills training, meditation, relaxation, deep breathing, exercise, journaling, time management, and goal setting (Murphy, 1984; Bond and Bunce, 2000; Alford *et al.*, 2005).

At this juncture, it is important to mention that given the wide array of stress management programs and outcome variables, there has been much debate as to which interventions, if any, are most effective. Some critics have argued that most studies on interventions are often inconclusive and based largely on methodologically weak research.

Meanwhile, the beginning of 21st century saw the emergence of a new movement, called 'positive psychology'. This model was based on the fact that most studies in the field of psychology were extensive focused on negative, pathological aspects of human functioning and behavior, while ignoring the fact that normal human naturally perceive life events not only negatively but positively (Pandey and Gaur, 2005).

The researchers in advocating for positive psychology therefore focused on the following:

- *subjective experiences*: well-being, contentment and satisfaction (from the past), hope and optimism (for the future); and flow and happiness (in the present).
- *Positive individual traits*: The capacity for love and vocation, courage, interpersonal skill, aesthetic sensibility, perseverance, forgiveness, originality, future mindedness, spirituality, high talent and wisdom.

- *Civic virtues* that motivate individuals towards better citizenship by promoting responsibility, nurturance, altruism, civility, moderation, tolerance and work ethic.

Alternatively, research in positive psychology rooted in positive mental health (PMH) and preventive stress management models is aimed at three levels of interventions. The *Primary prevention interventions* are designed to reduce, modify, or manage the intensity, frequency and/or duration of organizational demands and stressors to enhance health and reduce distress in people at work. The *Secondary prevention interventions* aim to reduce individuals' experience of the stress response. Meanwhile, the *Tertiary prevention interventions* were designed to minimize distress and provide therapy and improve the healing process from stressful events in organizations (Quick *et al*, 1998; Pandey and Gaur, 2005). Table 2 (in appendix section) illustrates the positive mental health (PMH) model while addressing the objectives of the intervention levels.

Accordingly, it is assumed that organization with 'positive mental health' provides a work environment to its individuals and teams that help them in maintaining their work-life balance and well-being while developing them into healthy personalities. Other implications of PMH include reduction in costs in terms of attrition, absenteeism, inefficient people and teams, occupational hazards and low productivity while maintaining productivity within the organization.

## Conclusion

The present work explored the subject of stress among nurses and approaches to effective stress management, notably, positive psychology. It also spotlights the implications of chronic stress to the expectations of high performance from nursing professional in relation to other components of the health system. This review is crucial as it exposes the issues on the impact of stress on organizational effectiveness from the perspective of the nursing professionals whose roles have been widely accepted as demanding to physical and mental well-being. Another significance of this review is on the need for more research into the effective coping strategies and stress management interventions for nurses. This provides many beneficial outcomes including optimized patient care.

It is also important to address stress within the working environment of many developing countries; many of whom are plagued by poor economic indices and high unemployment rate which have been shown to further heightens personal and workplace stress in healthcare organizations already threatened by shortage of professionals such as the nurses.

# References

Alford, W. K., Malouff, J. M., & Osland, K. S. (2005). Written emotional expression as a coping method in child protective services officers. International Journal of Stress Management, 12, 177–187.

Arthur, A. R. (2000). Employee assistance programmes: The emperor's new clothes of stress management? British Journal of Guidance and Counselling, 28, 549–559.

Bacharach, S.B., Bamberger, P., & Conley, S. (1991). Work home Conflict among Nurses and Engineers: Mediating the Impact of Role Stress on Burnout and Satisfaction at Work. Journal of Organizational Behaviour, 12, pp.39-53.

Barnett, R.C., Gareis, K.C., & Brennan, R.T. (1999). Fit as a Moderator of the Relationship between Work Hours and Burnout. Journal of Occupational Health Psychology, 4, pp.307-317.

Bedeian, A.G., Burke, B.G., & Moffett, R.G. (1998). Outcomes of Work-Family Conflict among Married Male and Female Professionals. Journal of Management, 14, pp.475-491.

Beehr, T.A., & Newman, J. (1978). Job Stress, Employee Health and Organizational Effectiveness: A Facet Analysis Model and Literature Review. Personnel Psychology, 31, pp.655-669.

Berber, N.; Lekovic, B. The impact of HR development on innovative performances in central and eastern European countries. Empl. Relat. 2018, 40, 762–786.

Bhagat, R.S. (1980). Effects of Personnel Life Stress, Upon Individual Performance of Effectiveness and Work Adjustment Processes within Orgnaizational Settings. James Mcken Cattel invited address delivered to the Division of Individual Organizational Psychology, American Psychological Association (J.R. Hackman, Chair), Montreal.

Bhagat, R.S. (1983). Effects of Stressful Life Events on Individual Performance Effectiveness and Work Adjustment Processes within Organizational Settings: A Research Model. Academy of Management Review, 84, pp.660-671.

Bhagat, R.S., McQuaid, S.J., Lindholm, H., & Segovis, J. (1985). Total Life Stress: A Multimedia Validation of the Construct and Its Effects on Organizationally Valued Outcomes and

Withdrawal Behaviors. Journal of Applied Psychology, 70, pp.202-214.

Bickford, M. (2005). Stress in the Workplace: A General Overview of the Causes, the Effects and the Solutions. Canadian Mental Health Association. retrieved from http://www.cmhanl.ca.

Billing, A.G., & Moos, R.H. (1982). Work Stress and the Stress-Buffering Roles of Works and Family Resources. Journal of Occupational Behaviour, 3, pp.215-232.

Bond, F. W., & Bunce, D. (2000). Mediators of change in emotion-focused and problem-focused worksite stress management interventions. Journal of Occupational Health Psychology, 5, 156–163.

Bonnie, S (2007) Job satisfaction , Work related stress and intentions to quit Scottish GPS, Report, National Primary Care Research and Development Centre, Williamson Building, University of Manchestor, Oxford Road, Manchestor.

Briner, R. (1999). Against the Grain. People Management, Sept., pp.32-41.

Burden, D.S. & Googins, B (1987). Boston University Balancing Job and Home Life Study. Boston University School of Social Work.

Burke, R.J., & Bradshaw, P. (1981). Occupational and Life Stress and the Family. Small Group Behaviour, 12, pp.329-375.

Burke, R.J., & Greeglass, E.R. (1999). Work Conflict, Spouse Support, and Nursing Staff Well-being During Organizational Structuring. Journal of Occupational Health Psychology, 4, pp.327-336.

Burke, R.J., & Weir, T. (1980). Coping with the Stress of Managerial Occupations. York University, Ontario.

Caplan, R.D. (1971). Organizational Stress and Individual Strain: A Social- Psychological Study of Risk Factors in Coronary Heart Disease Among Administrators, Engineers, and Scientists. Ann Arbor: Unpublished Doctoral Disseration, The University of Michigan.

Caplan, R.D. (1972). Organizational Stress and Individual Strain: A Social- Psychological Study of Risk Factors in Coronary

Heart Disease Among Administrators, Engineers, and Scientists. Dissertation Abstracts International, 32, 6706B – 6707B.

Caplan, R.D. (1983). Person-Environment Fit: Past, Present and Future. In C.L. Cooper (Ed.), Stress Research (pp.35-107). New York: Wiley.

Carranza, J.C. (1973). A Study of the Impact of Life Changes on High School Teacher Performance in Lansing School District as Measured by the Homes and Rahe Schedules of Recent Experiences. Dissertation Abstracts International, 33, 499A.

Chen, P.Y., & Spector, P.E. (1992). Relationships of Work Stressors with Aggression, Withdrawal, Theft and Substance Use: An Exploratory Study. Journal of Occupational and Organizational Psychology, September, pp.177-184.

Coleman, J.C., Morris, C.G., & Glares, A.C. (1987). Contemporary Psychology and Effective Behaviour (Sixth Ed.) Glenview IL: Scott, Foresman.

Dawkins, J.E., Depp., F. & Seltzar, N. (1985). Stress and the Psychiatry Nurse. Journal of Psychosocial Nursing, 23, 11, pp.9-15.

Diener, E. (1984). Subjective Well-being. Psychological Bulletin, 95, pp.542-575.

Dohrenwend, B.S., Krasnoff, L., Askenasy, A.R. & Dohrenwend, B.P. (1978). Exemplification of a Method for Scaling Life Events: The PERI Life Events Scale. Journal of Health and Social Behaviour, 19, pp.205-229.

Escartín, J.; Rodríguez-Carballeira, A.; Zapf, D.; Porrúa, C.; Martín-Peña, J. Perceived severity of various bullying behaviours at work and the relevance of exposure to bullying. Work Stress 2009, 23, 191–205.

Etzion, D. (1988). The Experience of Burnout and Work/non-Work Success in Male and Female Engineers: A Matched-Pairs Comparison. Human Resource Management, 27, pp.163-179.

Etzion, D., Eden, D., & Lapidot, Y. (1998). Relief from Job Stressors and Burnout: Reserve Service as a Respite. Journal of Applied Psychology, 83, pp.577-585.

Fried, Y.; Shirom, A.; Gilboa, S.; Cooper, C.L. The mediating effects of job satisfaction and propensity to leave on role stress-job performance relationships: Combining meta-analysis and structural equation modeling. In: From Stress to Wellbeing Volume 1; Palgrave Macmillan: London, UK, 2013; pp. 231–253.

Frone, M.R., Russell, M. & Cooper, M.L. (1992). Antecedents and Outcomes of Work- Family Conflict: Testing a Model of the Work-Family Interface. Journal of Applied Psychology, 77, pp.65-78.

Ganster, D.C., & Schaubroeck, J. (1991). Work Stress and Employee Health. Journal of Management, 17, pp.235-271.

Goff, S.J., Mount, M.K., & Jamison, R.L (1990). Employer supported child care, work/family conflict, and absenteeism: A field study, Personnel Psychology, 43, 793- 809.

Goldberger, L., & Breznitz, S (Eds). (1982). Handbook of stress and coping: Theoretical and clinical aspects New York: Free Press.

Gorgich E.A.C., Zare S., Ghoreishinia G., Barfroshan S., Arbabisarjou A., Yoosefia N. (2017). Job Stress and Mental Health Among the Nursing Staff in Educational Job Stress and Mental Health Among Nursing Staff of Educational Hospitals in South East Iran. Thrita. 2017 March; 6(1): e45421. doi: 10.5812/thrita.45421.

Greenhaus, J.H., & Parasuraman, S (1987). A w2ork-nonwork interactive perspective of stress and its consequences. In J.M Ivancevich & D C Ganster(Eds), Job stress: From theory to suggestion (pp 37-60), New York: Haworth.

Gupta, N., & Beehr, T.A (1979). Job stress and employee behaviour and Human Performance, 23, 373-387.

Hannigan B., Edwards D., Burnard, P., Coyle, D., & Fothergill, A. (2000) (a). Mental health nurses feel the strain. Mental Health Nursing.20,3,10-13.

Harris, P W. (1973). The relationship of life change to academic performance among selected college freshmen at varying levels of college readiness. Dissertation Abstracts International, 33, 6665A.

Hayness, S.G., Eaker, E.D., & Feinleib, M (1984). The effects of employment, family and job stress on coronary heart disease patterns in women, In E.B. Gold (Ed), The changing risk of disease in women: An epidemiological approach (pp. 37-48). Lexington, M.A: Health.

Hourani, L.L, Williams, T.V and Kriss, A.M (2006) Stress, Mental health and job performance among active duty military personnel. Military Medicine, September 2006.

House, J S (1983). Work stress and social support. Reading, M.A Addison – Wesley.

Ivancevich, J. M., Matteson, M. T., Freedman, S. M., & Phillips, J. S. (1990). Worksite stress management interventions. American Psychologist, 45, 252–261.

Jagdish & Srivastava, A.K (1983) Construction and Standardization of mental health inventory: A Pilot study Perspective in Psychological Researches, 6,35-37.

Johnson, J.H., & Sarason, I.G (1979) Recent developments in research on life stress. In V Hamilton and D.M Warburton (Eds.), Human stress and cognition: An information processing approach (pp.205-236) New York: Wiley.

Kahn, R.L ., & Quinn, R P (1970). Role Stress: A framework for analysis. In McLean (Ed.), Occupational mental health (pp.50-115), Chicago: Rand McNally.

Kanner, A., Kafry, D., & Pines, A (1978). Conspicuous in its absence: The lack of positive conditions as a source of stress. Journal of Human Stress, 4,33-39.

Karasek, R. (1979). Job demands, job decision latitude, and mental strain: Implications for job redesign. Administrative Science Quarterly, 24, 285–306.

Katic I., Kneževic T., Berber N., Ivaniševic A., Leber M. (2019).The Impact of Stress on Life, Working, and Management Styles:

How to Make an Organization Healthier? Sustainability, 11, 4026; doi:10.3390/su11154026.

Kaur. R., & and Chaddha., N.K (1988). Study of job stress with job involvement and job satisfaction. Indian Journal of Behaviour, 12,3,34-40.

Kelloway, E K., B.H., & Barham, L.(1999). The source, nature and direction of work and family conflict: A longitudinal investigation. Journal of Occupational Health Psychology, 4,337-346.

Kelloway, E.K., Gottlieb, B.H., & Barham, L, (1999). The source, nature, and direction of work and family conflict: A longitudinal investigation. Journal of Occupational Health Psychology, 4, 337-346.

Khodabaksh,A and Kolivand A (2006) Stress and Job satisfaction among Airforce Military Pilots. Journal of Social Sciences, Vol.2, No.4: 121-124.

Krantz, D S., Glass, D.C., Contrada, R., & Miller, N (1981). Behaviour and health. New York: Social Science Research Council.

Krantz, D.S., Glass, D.C., Contrada, R., & Miller, N (1981). Behaviour and health, New York: Social Science Research Council.

Kumari, P., Vishwavidyalaya, G. K. and Mishra, R. (2009) 'Effect of Job Stress and Personal Life Stress on Mental Health and Job Outcomes of Medical Professionals. doi: 10.2139/ssrn.1437409.

Kupriyanov, R., Zhdanov R. (2014). The Eustress Concept: Problems and Outlooks. World Journal of Medical Sciences, 11(2), 179-185. doi:10.5829/idosi.wjms.2014.11.2.8433

Lazarus, R. S. and Launier, R. (1978). Stress-related transactions between person and environment. In L A Pervin and M Lewis (Eds), (1978). Perspectives in Interactional Psychology. pp. 287–327.

Lazarus, R.S., & Folkman, S (1984) Stress appraisal and coping. New York: Springer.

Leiter, M.P.., & Schaufeli, W.B. (1996). Consistency of the burnout construct across occupations. Anxiety, Stress and Coping, 9,229-243.

Lindo, J.L.M., McCaw – Binns, A; La Grenade, J. Jackson, M and Shearer, D.E (2008). Mental well being of doctors and nurses in two hospitals in Kingston , Jamaica, West Indian Medical Journal, Vo 55, No.3.

Maslach, C., & Schaufeli, W.B (1993), Historical and conceptual development of burnout. In W.B. Schaufeli C. Maslach & T.Marck (Eds), Professional burnout: Recent developments in theory and research (pp.1-16). Washington DC: Taylor & Francis.

Matteson, M.T., & Ivancevich, J.M (1987). Controlling work stress: San Francisco, London: Jpssey-Bass publishers.

Melchior, M., Caspi, A., Milne, B.J., Danese, A., Poulton, R. & Moffitt, T.E. (2007). Work stress precipitates depression and anxiety in young, working women and men. Psychological Medicine. 37(8). p. 1119-1129. doi: 10.1017/S0033291707000414.

Mohammad M A (2014). Occupational stress and its consequences: Implications for health policy and management. Leadersh. Health Serv. 27, 224–239.

Mottowidlo, S.J., & Packard, J.S. (1986). Occupational stress: Its causes and consequefor job performance. Journal of Applied Psychology, 71, 618-629.

Moustaka E., Constantinidis T.C. (2010). Sources and effects of Work-related stress in nursing. Health Science Journal, 4(4): 210–216.

Murphy LR, Sauter SL. Work organization interventions: state of knowledge and future directions. Soc Prev Med. 2004; 49:79–86.

Murphy, L. R. (1984). Occupational stress management: A review and appraisal. Journal of Occupational Psychology, 57, 1–15.

Nelson D., Cooper C.L. (2007) Positive Organizational Behavior. Sage Publications; London, United Kingdom. pp. 44-56.

Nelson, D.L., Simmons B.L. (2011). Health Psychology and Work Stress: A More Positive Approach. In Handbook of Occupational Health Psychology. Campbell Quick, J. & Tetrick, L.E. editors. American Psychological association. Washington; DC. USA. pp. 55-74.

Pandey, S. and Gaur, S. (2005). "A Positive Mental Health Model for Stress Management Interventions in Organizations: Insights from Positive Psychology", presented at 92nd Indian Science Congress, organized by Indian Science Congress Association, Nirma University, Ahmedabad and National Institute of Occupational Health, Ahmedabad, January 3-7, 2005.

Pestonjee, D.M (1973) Organizational structures and job attitudes. Calcutta: Minerva Associates.

Pestonjee, D.M., & Singh, A.P (1978). Performance Rating Scale, Varanasi: Abhishek Publications.

Pleck, J.H (1989). Family-supportive employer policies and men's participation: A perspective. Unpublished manuscript.

Popov, B.; Popov, S. Gender Differences in Experiencing Occupational Stress. Primenjenapsihologija 2011, 2, 179– 195.

Quick, J. D.; Quick, J. C. and Nelson, D. L. (1998). The theory of preventive stress management in organizations. In Cary L. Cooper (Ed.), Theories of Organizational Stress. New York: Oxford University Press.

Rice, R.W., Near, J.P., & Hunt, R.G (1980). The job satisfaction/life satisfaction relationship: A review of empirical research. Basic and Applied Social Psychology, 1,37-64.

Robet, A.B. (1986) Behaviour in Organization (2nd Ed.,) Boston: Allyn and Bacon. Ryan, D., & Quayle, E. (1999). Stress in psychiatry nursing: Fact or fiction? Nursing Standard,14,8,32-35.

Sarason, I.G. Johnson, J.H & Siegel, J.M (1978). Assessing the impact of life changes: Development of the life experience survey. Journal of Consulting and Clinical Psychology, 46,932-946.

Schoonmaker,A (1969). Anxiety and the executive. New York : The American Management Association.

Schuler, R.J (1980). Definition and conceptualization of stress in organizations. Organizational Behaviour and Human Performance, 25, 184-215.

Schultz, D. (1977). Growth psychology: Models of the healthy personality. New York: Van Nostrand, Reinhold.

Semmer NK. Job stress interventions and the organization of work. Scand J WorK Environ Health 2006;32(6, special issue):515–527.

Shinn, M., Wong., N.W., Simko, P.A., & Oritz – Torres, B. (1989). Promoting the well- being of working parents. Coping, social support and flexible hob schedules. American Journal of Community Psychology, 17,31-55.

Shirom, A. (1989). Burnout in work organizations. In C.L. Cooper & I Robertson (Eds.), International review of industrial and organizational psychology, (pp.25-48). New York: Wiley.

Siegrist, J. Chronic psychosocial stress at work and risk of depression: Evidence from prospective studies. Eur. Arch. Psychiatry Clin. Neurosci. 2008, 258 (Suppl. 5), 115–119.

Srivastava, O.N., & Bhatt, V.K (1973). Mental ill-health questionnaire. An unpublished standardized measure of mental health. Department of Psychology, Banaras Hindu University.

Stains, G.L (1980). Spillover versus compensation: A review of the literature on the relationship between work and non-work Human Relations, 33, 111-129.

Sullivan, P.J (1993) Occupational stress in psychiatry nursing. Journal of Advanced Nursing, 18, 591-601.

Tehrani N, Ayling L (2009). Work-related stress. CIPD Stress at work, June 2009. http://www.cipd.co.uk/subjects/health/stress/stress.htm, Accessed :17-11-2021.

Torrence, E.P (1965). Mental health and consecutive behaviour. Belmont California: Wadsworth.

Vinokur, A., & Selzer, M. (1975). Desirable versus undesirable life events: Their relationship to stress and mental distress, Journal of Personality and Social Psychology, 66, 297-333.

Westman, M., & Eden, D (1997). Effects of vacation on job stress and burnout: Relief and fade-out. Journal of Applied Psychology, 82, 516-527.

Zander, A., & Quinn, R.P (1962) The social environment and mental health: A review of past research at the Institute ofSocial Research. Journal of Social Issues, 18,48-66.

Zohar, D (1997). Predicting burnout with a hassle based measure of role demands. Journal of Organizational Behaviour , 18,101-115.

# Appendix

**Table 1: The PMH Model** (adopted from Pandey and Gaur, 2005)

| INTERVENTION LEVELS/INTERVENTION STAGES | INDIVIDUAL | TEAM | ORGANIZATION |
|---|---|---|---|
| **Primary** | Goal setting; Lifestyle management; Managing the work environment; Managing perception of stress | Goal setting; Role analysis; Participative management; Partnering; Team competency assessment | Social support; Career development; task and job redesign |
| **Secondary** | Relaxation training; Emotional outlets; Physical fitness/nutrition | Team building; Role negotiations; Quality circles; Survey feedback; Education & training; Appreciations and concerns exercise | Diagnostic activities ; Relationship management; Improving organizational communication; Confrontation of macro-organizational issues |
| **Tertiary** | Medical care; Psychological counseling; Behavioral, therapy; Psychological therapy | Medical care; Psychological counseling; Behavioral, therapy; Psychological therapy | Organizational transformational activities; Diversity programs |

# YOUR KNOWLEDGE HAS VALUE

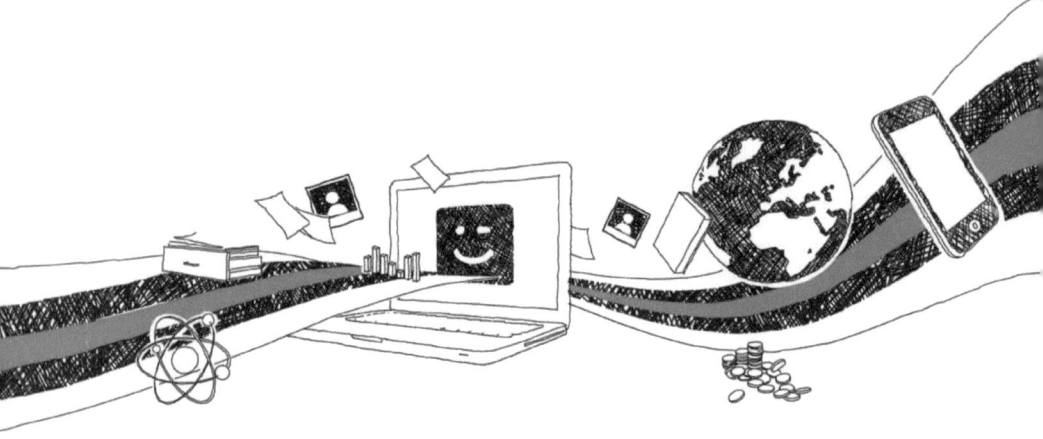

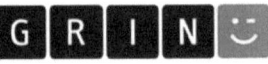